1950s TV Stars
MEMORY LANE

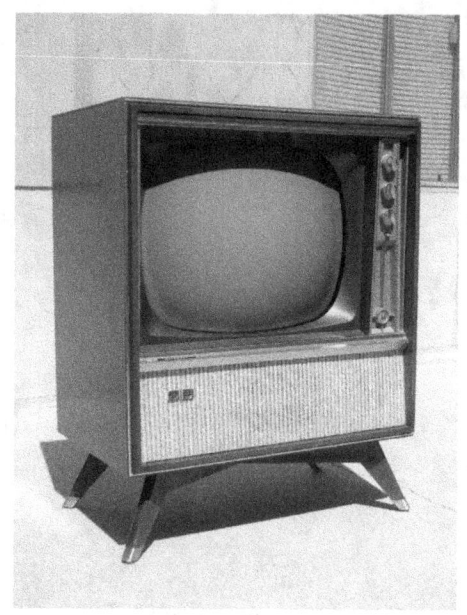

Compiled by Hugh Morrison

Montpelier Publishing

London

Cover pictures

Front (clockwise from left): Raymond Burr (Perry Mason).
Phil Silvers (Sergeant Bilko)
Howdy Doody
Lucille Ball and Desi Arnaz

Back: Clockwise from top: George Reeves as Superman.
The Honeymooners.
Rin Tin Tin.
Eddie 'Rochester' Anderson.

ISBN: 9781092560924

Published in Great Britain by Montpelier Publishing, London.

Printed and distributed by Amazon.

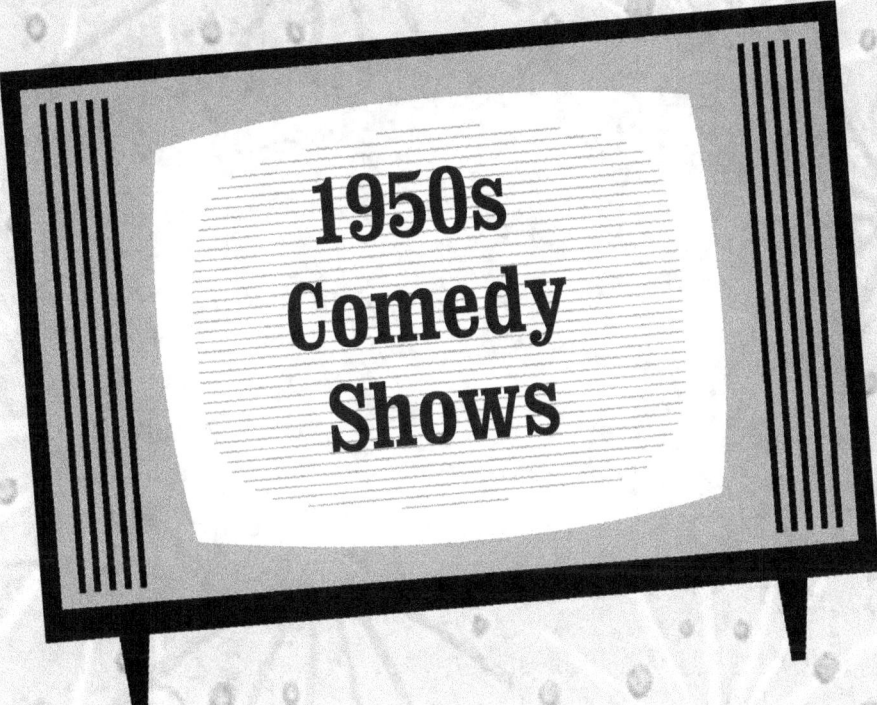

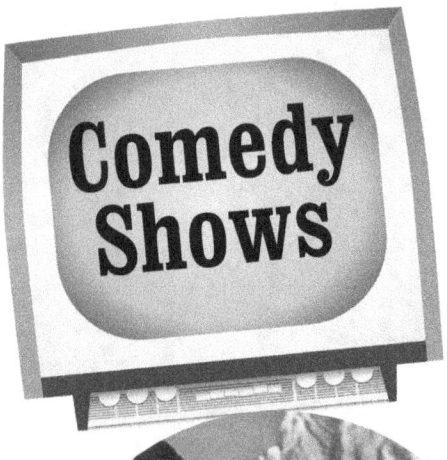

Comedy Shows

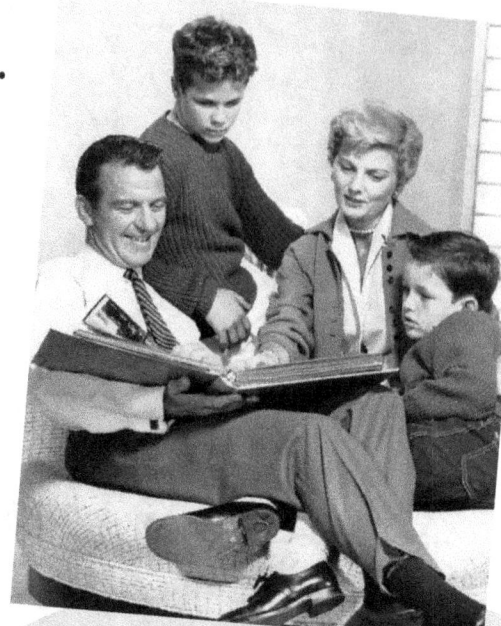

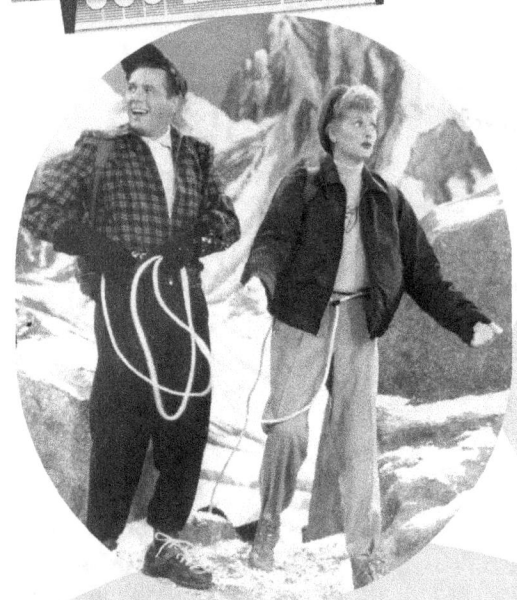

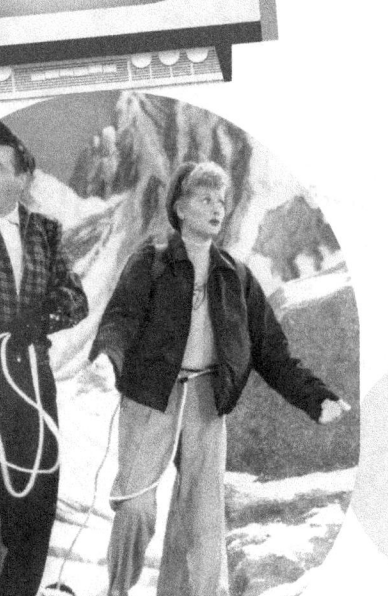

Leave it to Beaver
1957-1963

This family comedy revolved around the school and home life of Beaver Cleaver, his brother Wally and parents June and Ward.

I Love Lucy
1951-1957

Desi Arnaz and Lucille Ball starred as New York couple Ricky and Lucille Ricardo with their son, Ricky Jr.

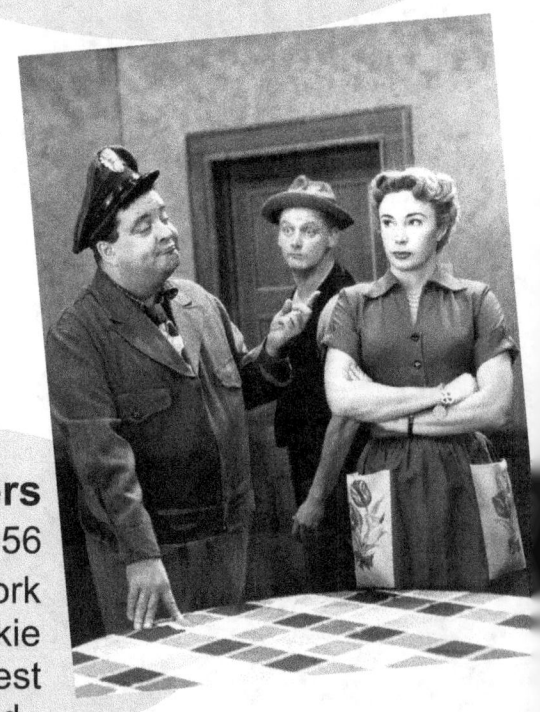

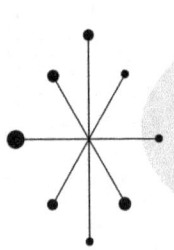

The Honeymooners
1955-1956

Classic comedy about New York bus driver Ralph (Jackie Gleason), his wife Alice and best friend Ed.

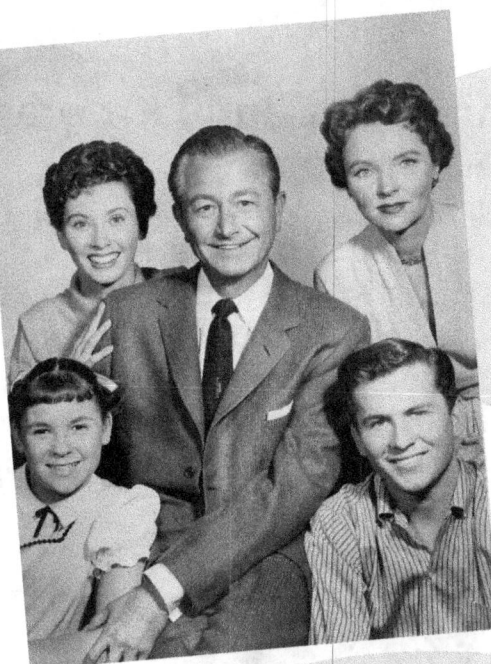

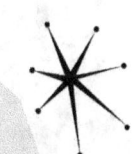

Father Knows Best
1954-1960

Popular family comedy about James and Margaret Anderson and their three children, Betty James and Kathy.

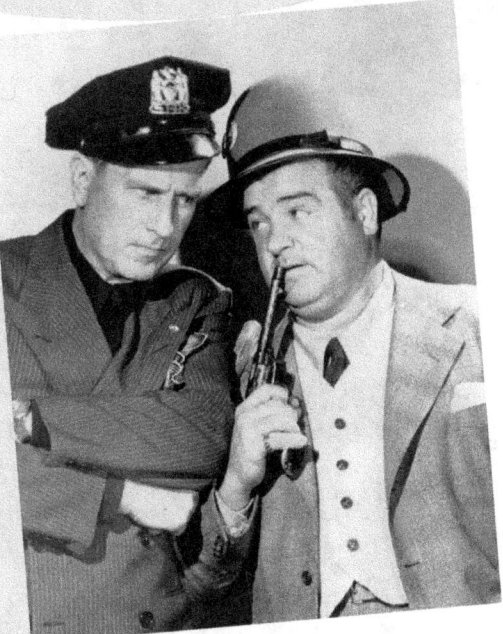

The Abbott and Costello Show
1952-1954

The TV adventures of vaudeville and movie comedians Bud Abbott (left) and Lou Costello. Lou's catchphrase was 'I'm a bad boy!'

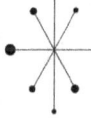

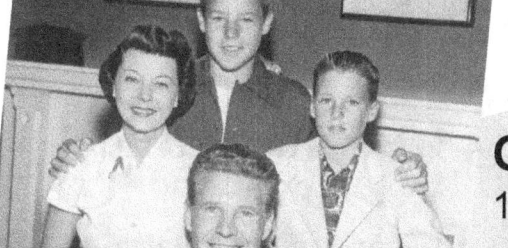

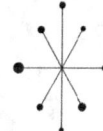

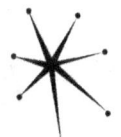

Ozzie and Harriet
1952-1966

The first TV comedy to run for more than ten years, this show featured Californian couple Ozzie and Harriet Nelson and their sons David and Ricky.

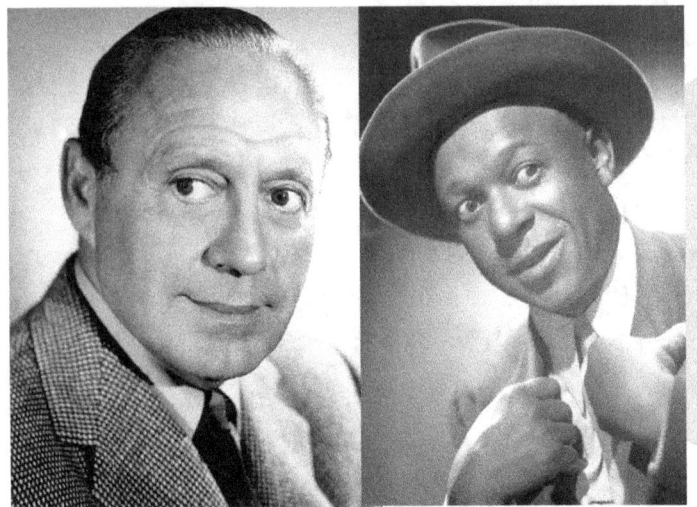

The Jack Benny Program
1950-1965
This hilarious show portrayed the comic capers of vaudeville star Jack Benny (left) and his valet, Rochester, played by Eddie Anderson. Benny's catchphrase was simply 'Well!'

The Phil Silvers Show
1955-1959
Originally titled *You'll Never Get Rich*, the show starred Phil Silvers as Sergeant Bilko, a wisecracking gambler always one step ahead of his senior officer, Colonel Hall.

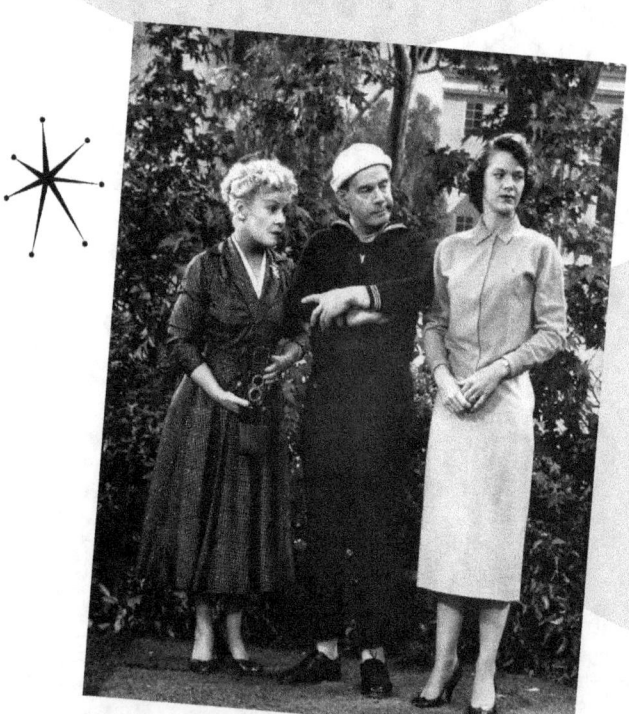

December Bride
1954-1959
This comedy, starring Spring Byington, centered on the life of Lily Ruskin, a sprightly widow seeking love with the help of her daughter Ruth and son-in-law Matt.

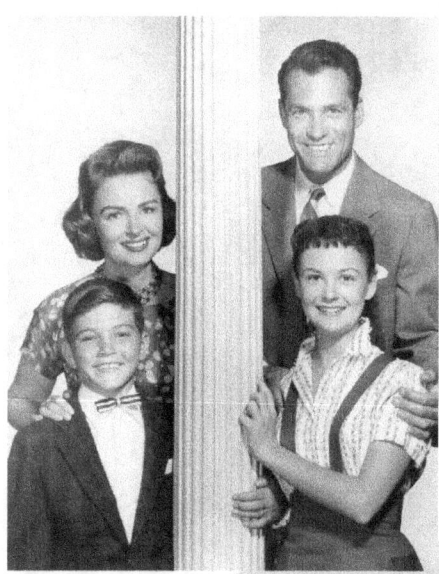

The Donna Reed Show
1958-1966

Starring Donna Reed as Donna Stone, a doctor's wife, this family comedy went on to become one of the most popular US TV sitcoms and launched the hit song, *Johnny Angel*.

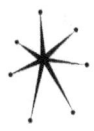

Dennis the Menace
1959-1963

Trouble-prone kid Dennis Mitchell was always getting into scrapes, much to the annoyance of his parents Henry and Alice, and neighbour George Wilson.

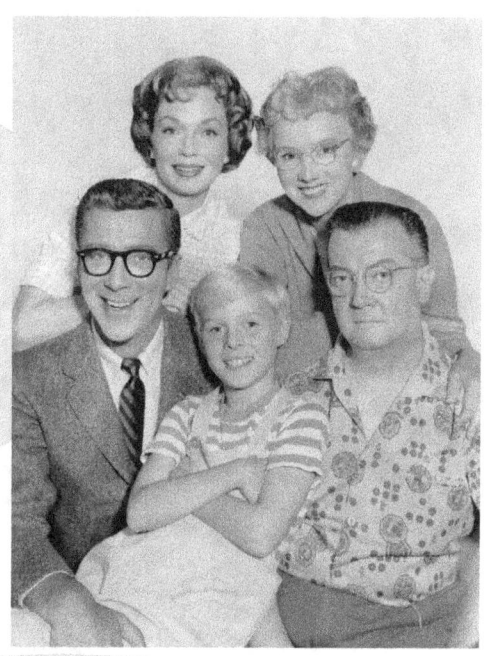

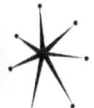

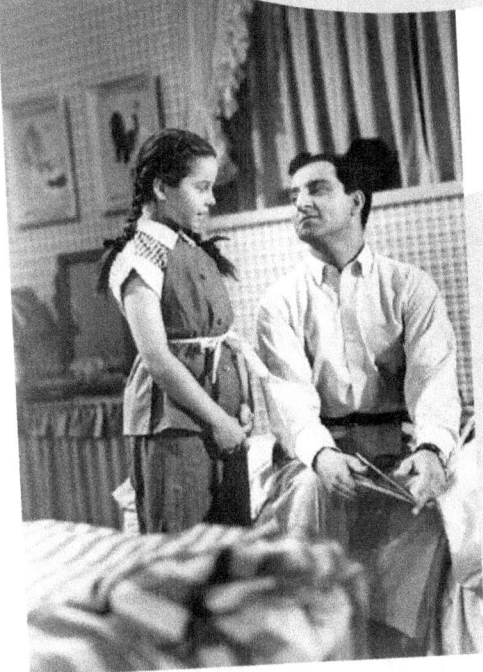

Make Room For Daddy
1953-1957

Also titled *The Danny Thomas Show*, this comedy was about the troubled home life of comedian Danny Williams (played by Danny Thomas), his wife Margaret, daughter Terry and son Rusty.

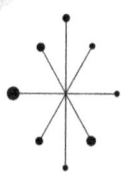

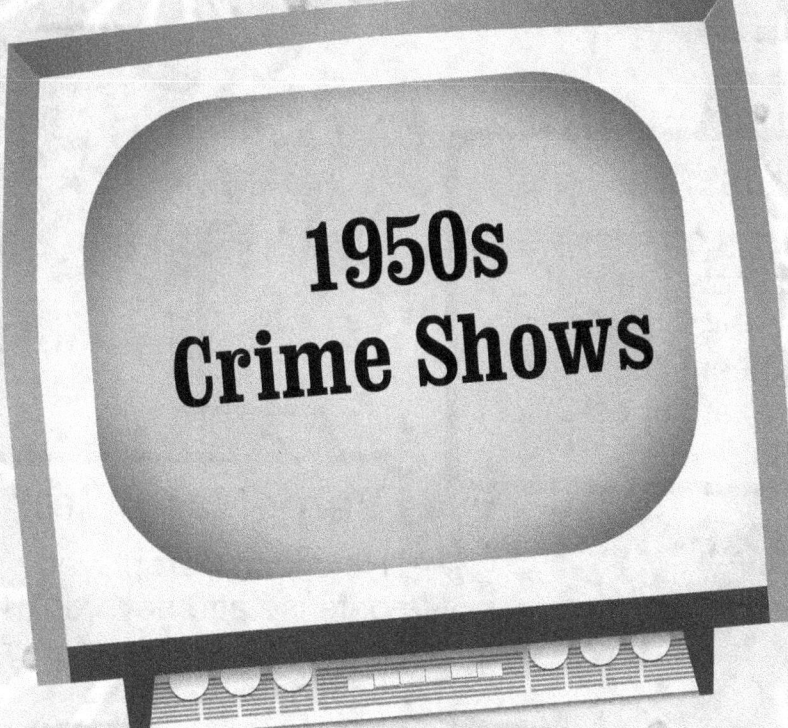

1950s
Crime Shows

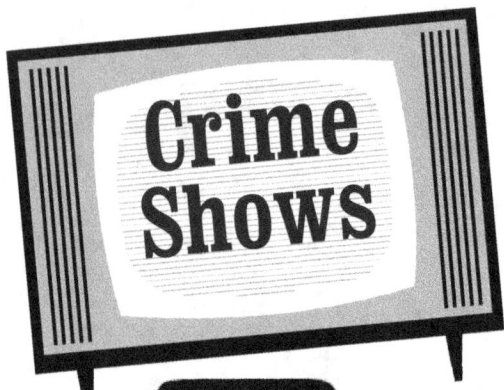

Crime Shows

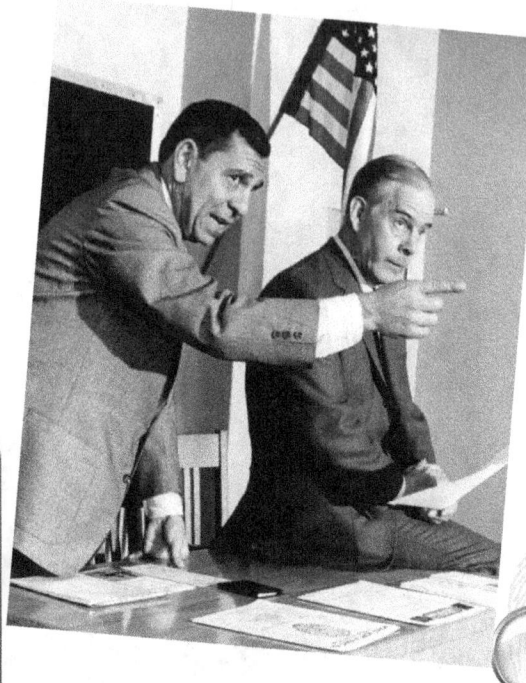

Dragnet 1951-1959

Long running Los Angeles-based cop show *Dragnet* starred Jack Webb *(above, left)* as Sergeant Joe Friday and Ben Alexander as Officer Frank Smith.

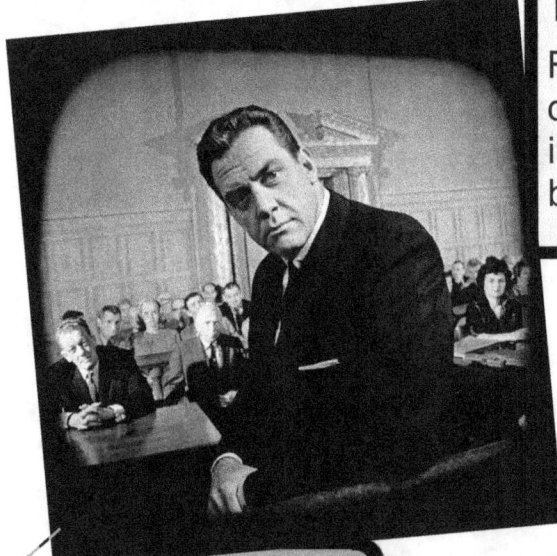

Perry Mason 1957-1966

Raymond Burr played defense attorney Perry Mason in this long-running courtroom based crime series.

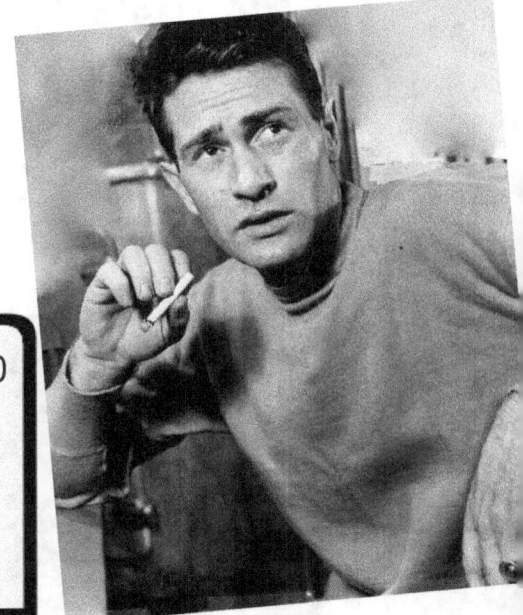

Mike Hammer 1958-1960

The tough New York private eye Mike Hammer was played by Darren McGavin with Bart Burns as Captain Chambers.

Peter Gunn 1958-1960

Peter Gunn, played by Craig Stevens, was a sharp dressed, jazz-loving private eye helped by his girlfriend Edie (Lola Hart).

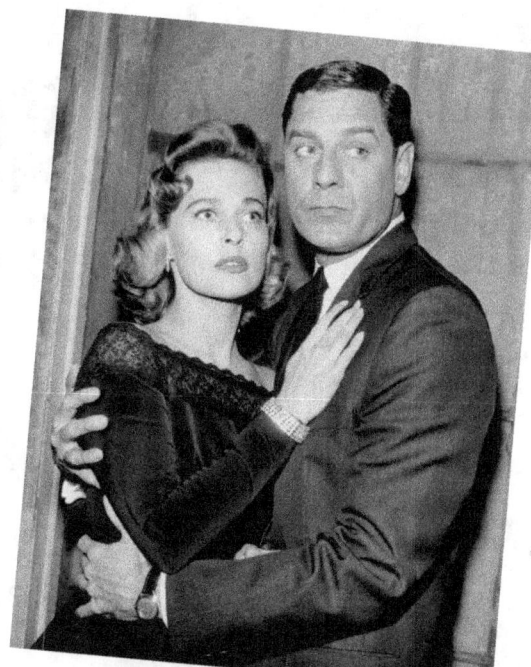

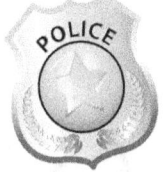

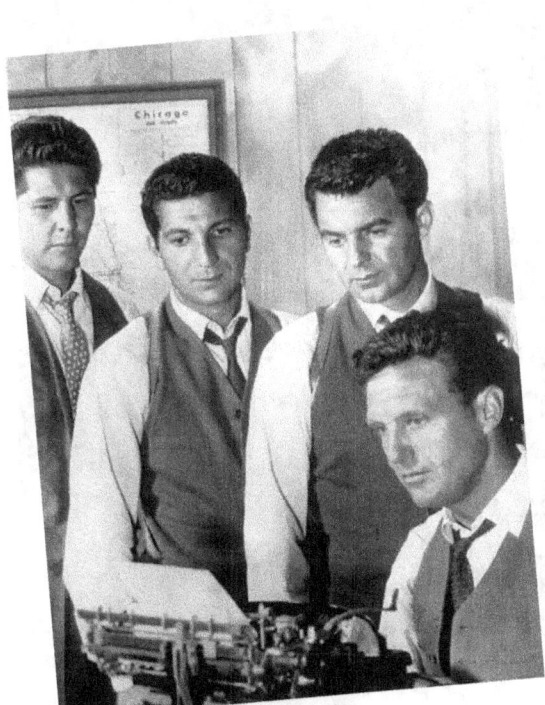

The Untouchables 1959-1963

Set in the 1920s, this show told the story of prohibition agents fighting against the Mob and Al Capone. It was based on the true life story of FBI agent Eliot Ness.

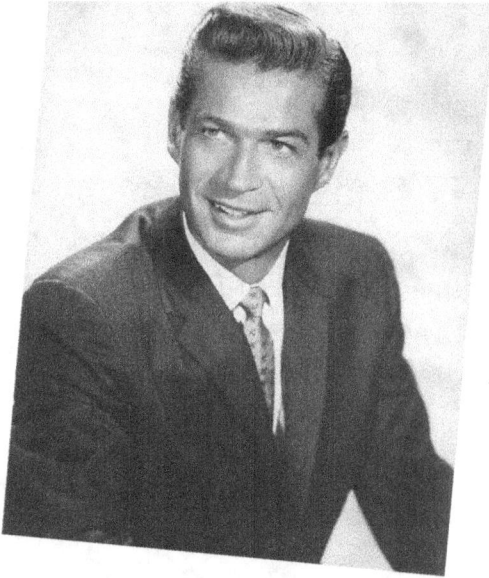

Ellery Queen 1950-1959

George Nader played Ellery Queen, the Harvard-educated, gentlemanly private investigator based in a large mansion in New York City.

Hawaiian Eye 1959-1963

Anthony Eisley played Tracy Steele, a suave private detective based in the Hawaiian Village Hotel in Honolulu, Hawaii.

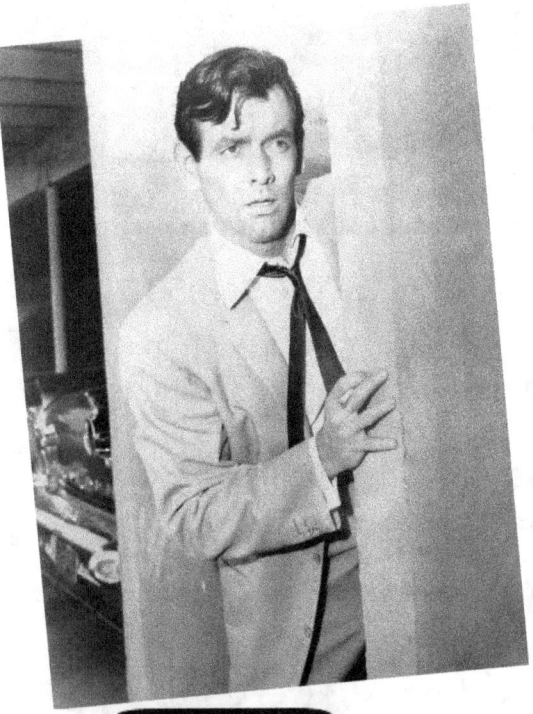

Richard Diamond, Private Detective 1957-1959

Richard Diamond, played by David Janssen, was a smooth talking, charming private investigator based in glamorous Hollywood.

77 Sunset Strip 1958-1964

77 Sunset Strip, Hollywood, was the address of Bailey and Spencer, private detectives. Efrem Zimbalist Jr *(right)* played Bailey and Roger Smith played Spencer.

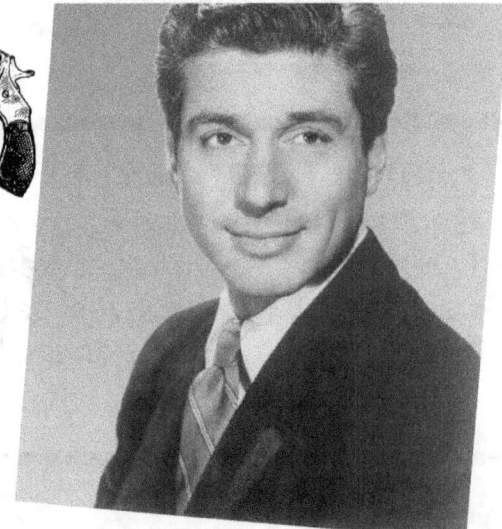

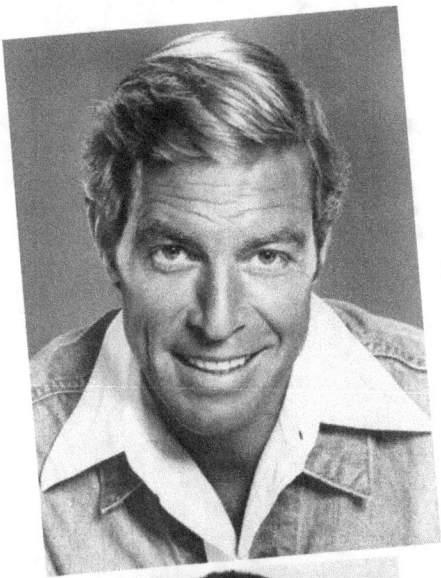

The Naked City 1958-1963

A documentary-style police drama series starring James Franciscus *(left)* as Detective Jimmy Halloran. The show always ended with the words 'There are eight million stories in the naked city; this has been one of them'.

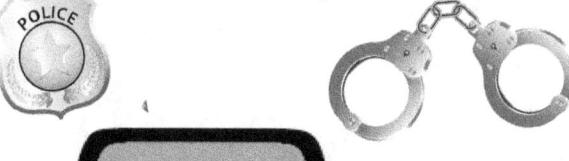

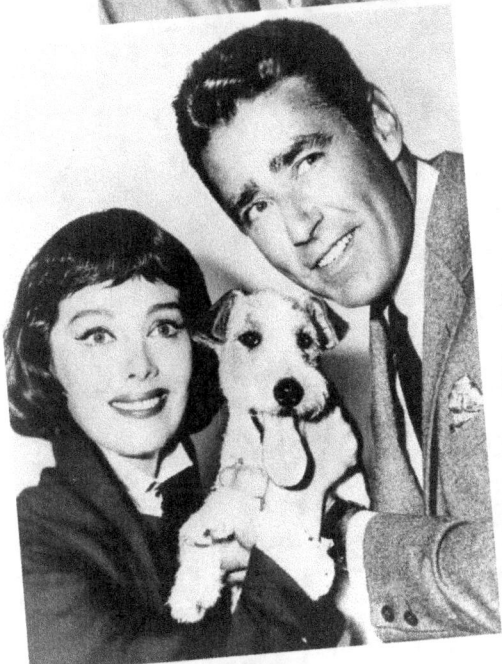

The Thin Man 1957-1959

This show starred Peter Lawford and Phyllis Kirk as amateur detectives Nick and Nora Charles with their dog, Asta. Nora was one of the first female detectives on TV.

Mr and Mrs North 1952-1954

Mr and Mrs North were wealthy socialites who also worked as private detectives. They were played by Richard Denning and Barbara Britton.

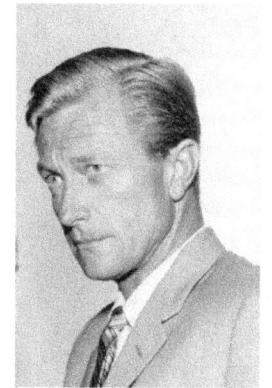
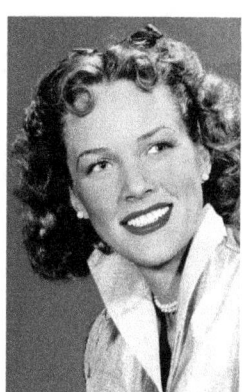

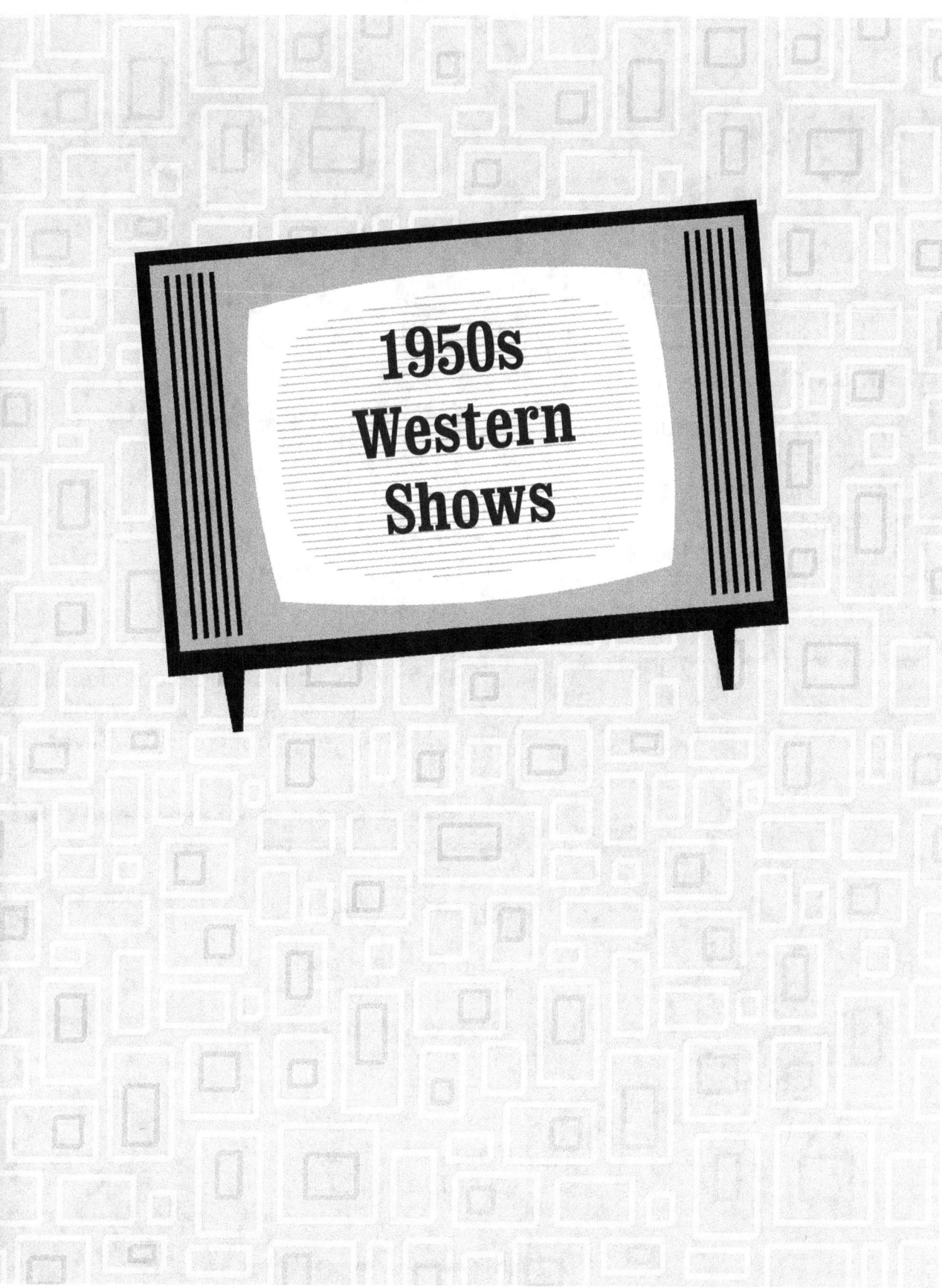

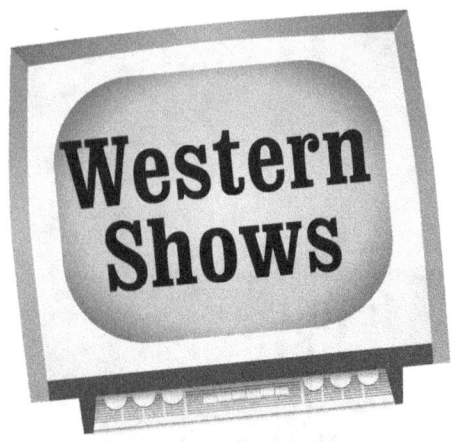

Western Shows

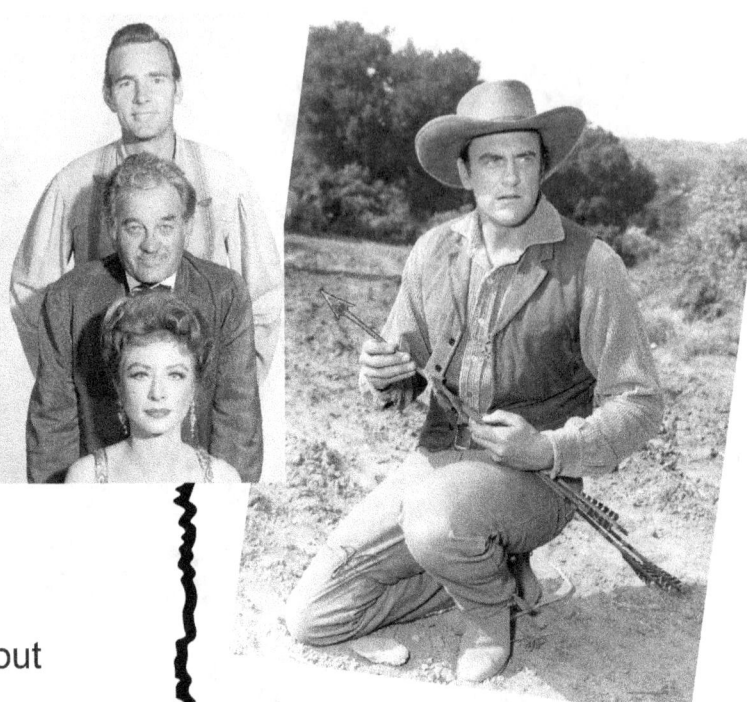

Gunsmoke 1955-1975

One of the most popular and long running US TV shows, *Gunsmoke* was about the adventures of Marshall Matt Dillon and his friends Chester, Doc Adams and Miss Kitty in Dodge City, Kansas.

The Lone Ranger 1949-1957

Clayton Moore *(left)* starred as the masked Lone Ranger with Jay Silverheels as his Indian companion, Tonto. Each episode ended with the Lone Ranger shouting 'Hi Yo Silver, Away!'

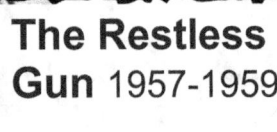

The Restless Gun 1957-1959

John Payne *(right)* played wandering cowboy Vint Bonner in this popular show.
The show's theme song was 'I Ride With The Wind'.

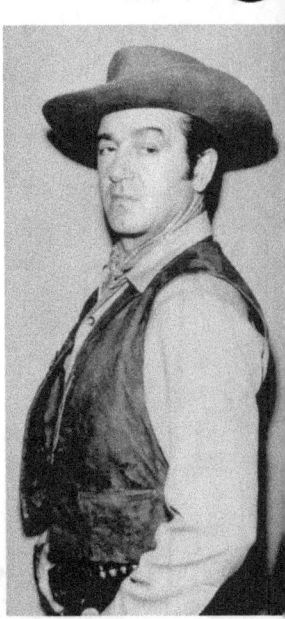

The Life and Legend of Wyatt Earp 1955-1961

This was the first prime-time US TV western show, and starred Hugh O'Brian *(right)* as frontier marshal Wyatt Earp.

Cheyenne 1955-1963

This was the first hour long drama show on US TV and featured Clint Walker as Cheyenne Brodie, a cowboy raised by Cheyenne Indians after his parents' death.

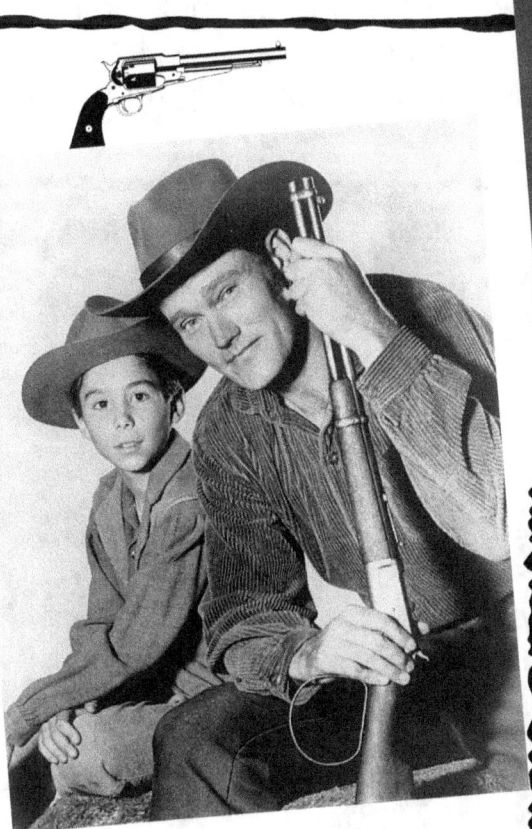

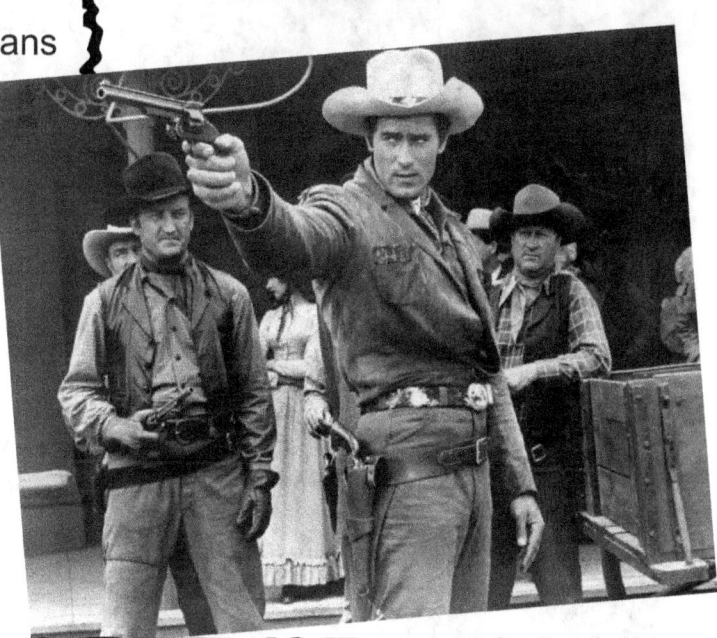

The Rifleman 1958-1963

Well known footballer Chuck Connors played rancher and crack shot Lucas McCain with Johnny Crawford as his son, Mark. Each episode opened with McCain firing his Winchester repeating rifle.

Bonanza 1959-1973

NBC's longest running western told the story of the Cartwright ranching family from Virginia City, Nevada. Lorne Greene *(right)* played the head of the family, Ben Cartwright.

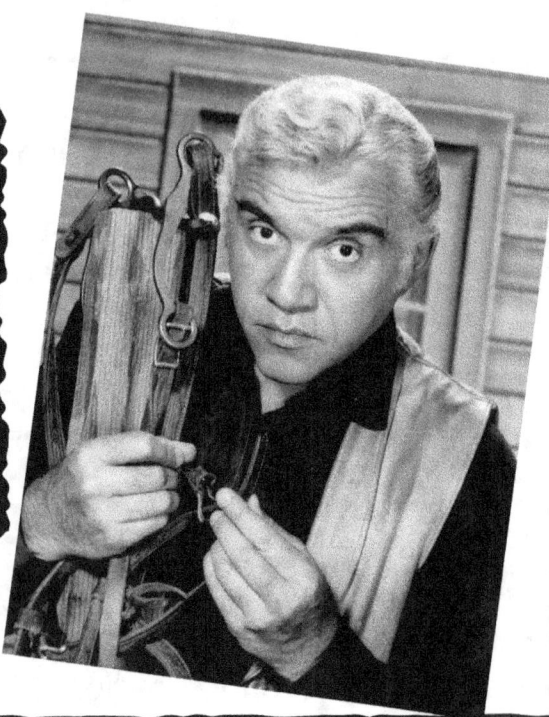

Maverick 1957-1962

James Garner *(left)* played wise-cracking card-sharp Bret Maverick who, with his brother Bart, traveled the West in search of big winnings.

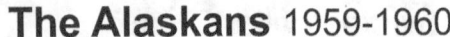

The Alaskans 1959-1960

British actor Roger Moore (who later played James Bond) starred as Silky Harris, a confidence trickster in the Yukon Gold Rush of the 1890s.

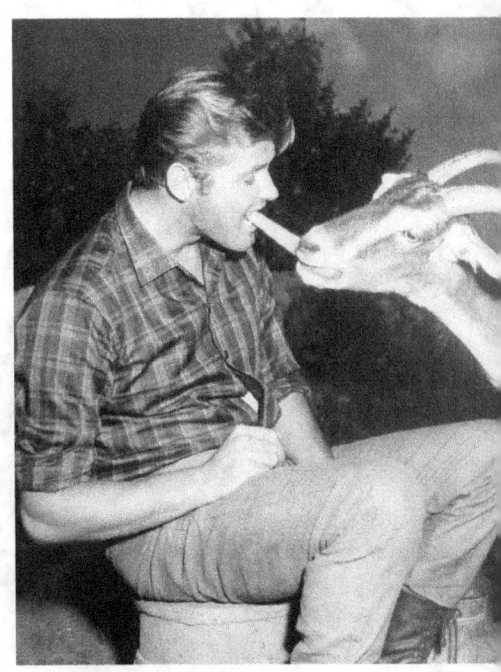

Colt 45 1957-1960

Wayde Preston *(right)* played undercover government agent Christopher Colt, posing as a pistol salesman while fighting crime in the Wild West.

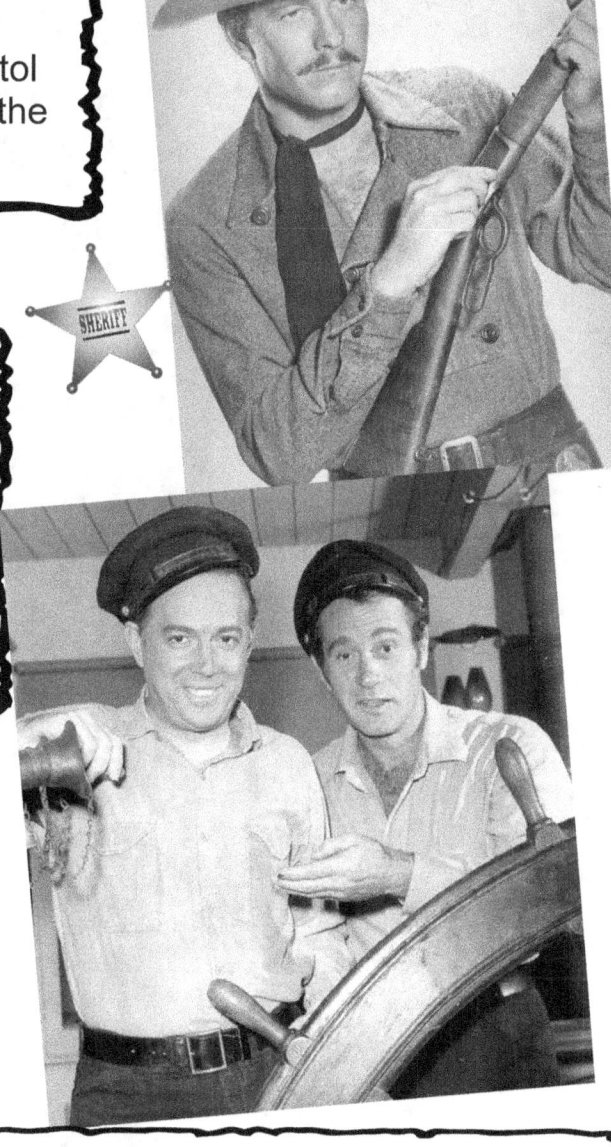

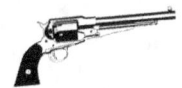

Riverboat 1959-1961

This show was about the adventures of a riverboat crew on the Mississippi and Ohio Rivers. Starring Darren McGavin *(far right)* as Captain Brad Turner, the show was set earlier than most westerns, in the 1840s.

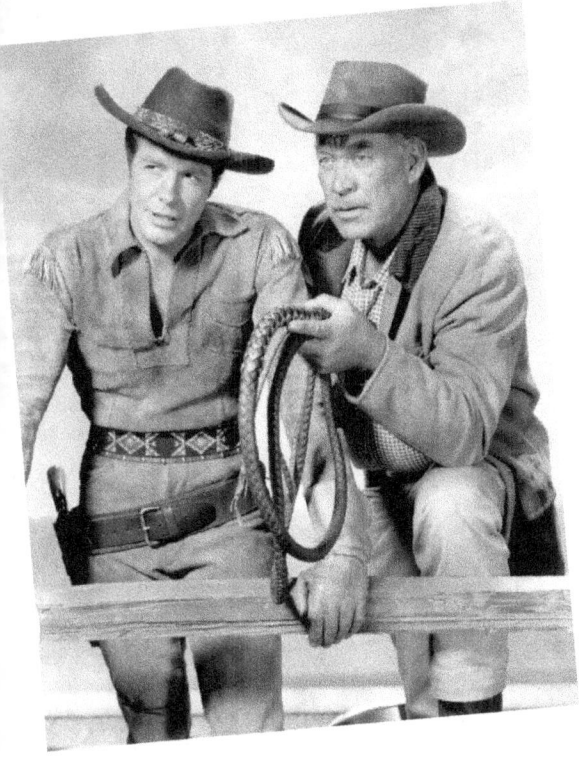

Wagon Train 1957-1965

The exciting story of a wagon train travelling from Missouri to California, starring Ward Bond *(left)* as Major Seth Adams and Robert Horton *(far left)* as Flint McCollough.

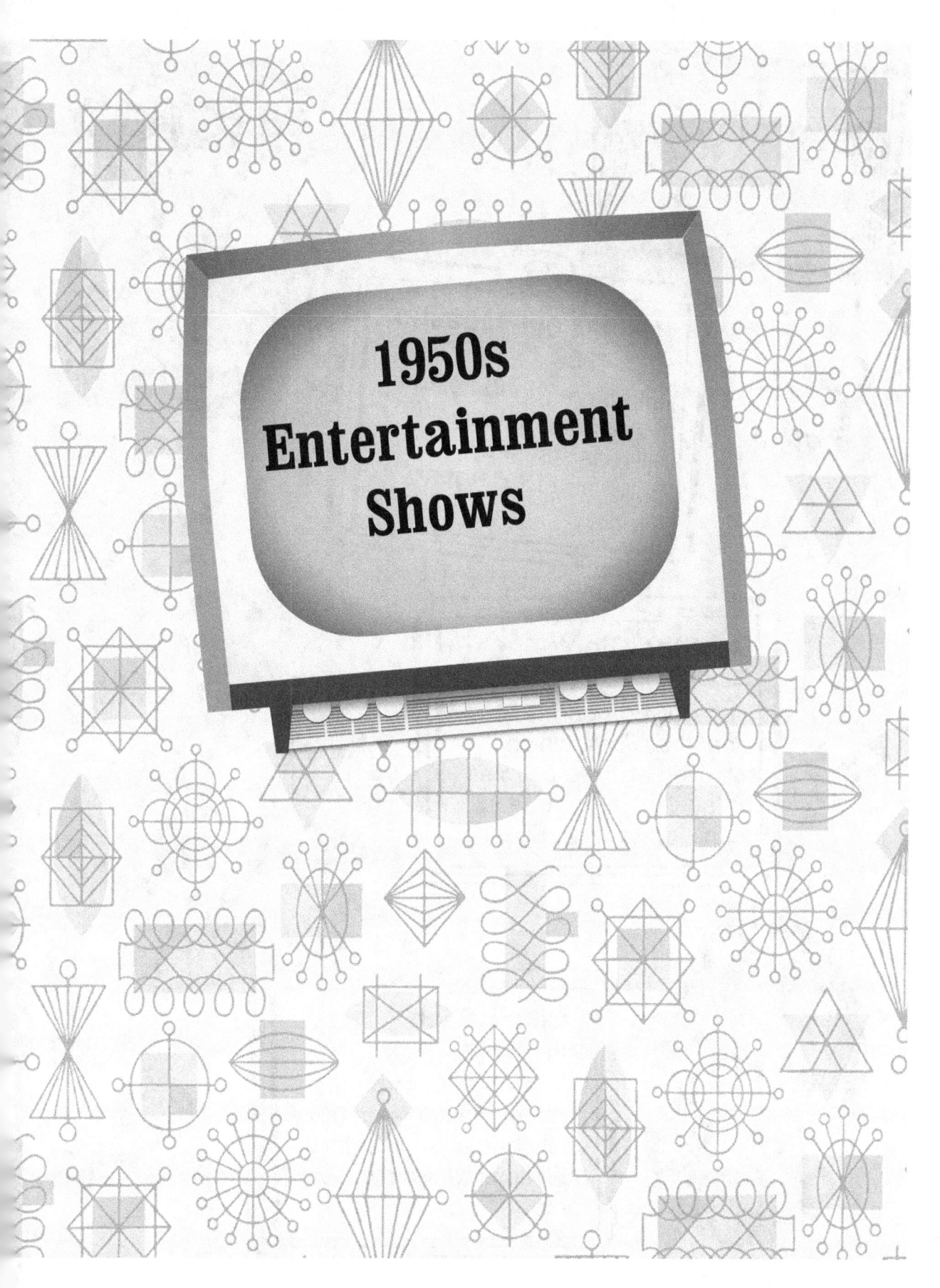

1950s Entertainment Shows

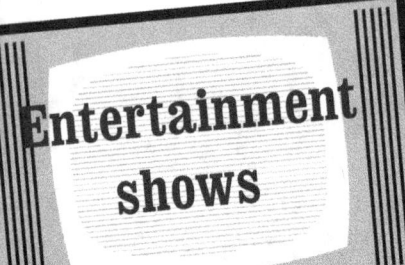

Entertainment shows

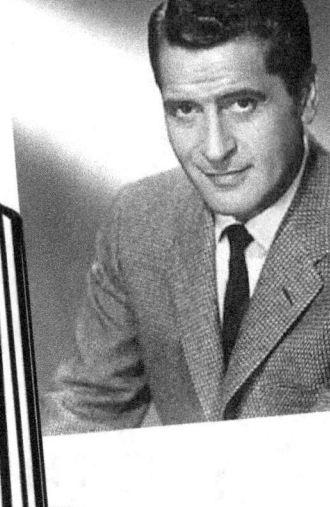

? ? ?

The $64,000 Question
1955-1958

Hal March *(right)* hosted this popular quiz show with assistants Lynn Dollar and Dr Bergen Evans.

Beat the Clock
1950-1961

Bud Colyer *(right)* hosted *Beat the Clock*, which involved married couples or families taking part in stunts to win big prizes.

$$$

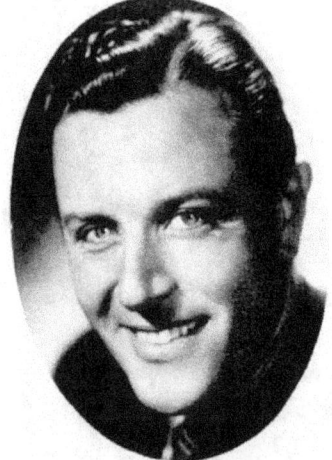

Strike it Rich
1951-1958

Hosted by Warren Hull *(left)*, contestants on this show had to answer four questions to win money for a good cause.

$$$
$$$

The Price is Right
1956-1965

This show was hosted by Bill Cullen *(right)* who invited the audience to win prizes by guessing their correct price.

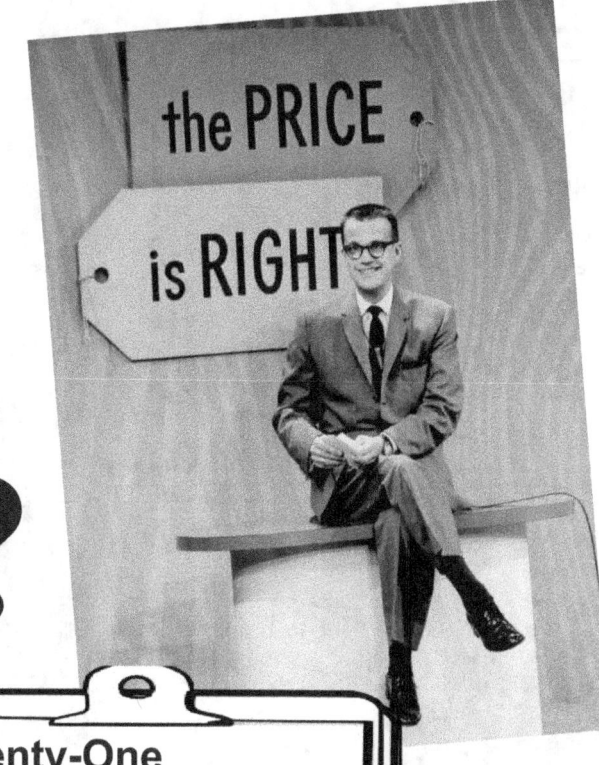

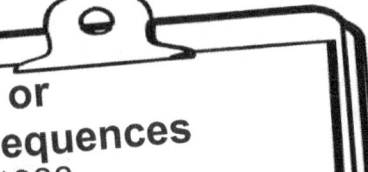

Twenty-One
1956-1958

In this quiz show, Jack Barry *(far left)* asked 21 questions to contestants who sat in 'isolation booths'.

$$$
$$$

Truth or Consequences
1950-1988

Bob Barker *(right)* was one of several presenters on this long-running quiz show where contestants had to carry out zany stunts.

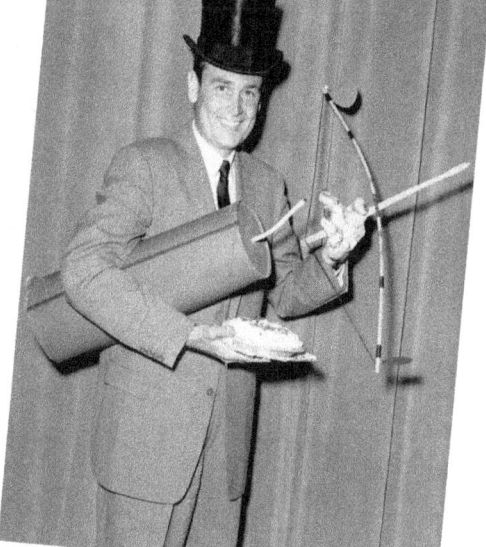

This is Your Life
1952-1961

Ralph Edwards *(right, with guest Lilian Roth)* hosted this show which took celebrity guests by surprise and told their life story.

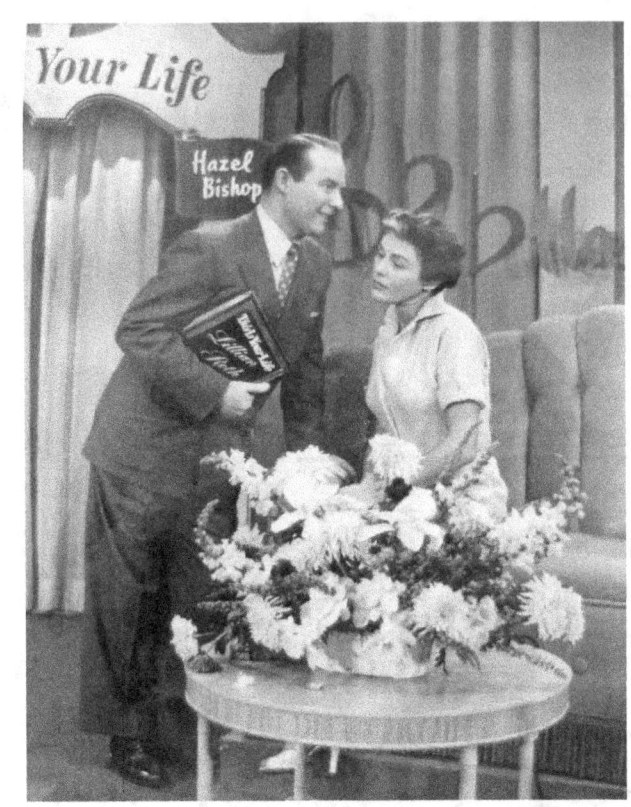

The George Burns & Gracie Allen Show
1950-1958

A scripted 'real life' entertainment show featuring veteran vaudeville comedians George Burns and Gracie Allen.

The Garry Moore Show
1950-1967

Garry Moore, Carol Burnett and Durward Kirby hosted this long running music and comedy sketch variety show.

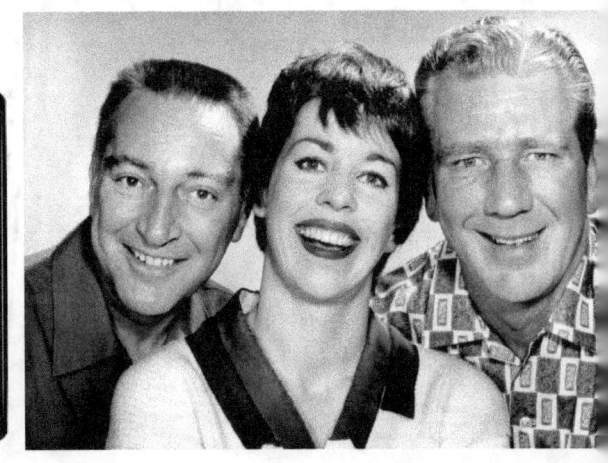

The Tonight Show
1954-present

This long running talk show on NBC was presented in the 1950s by Steve Allen and then Jack Paar *(right, interviewing Senator John F Kennedy in 1959).*

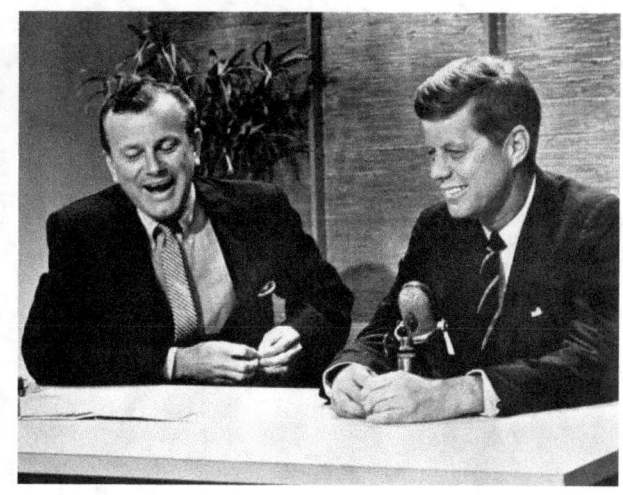

The Ed Sullivan Show
1948-1971

In this show, originally called *Toast of the Town*, host Ed Sullivan *(left)* introduced the top stars of stage, screen and music every Sunday night on CBS.

The Jackie Gleason Show
1952-1970

One of the most popular shows of the 1950s, featuring comedian Jackie Gleason *(right, with dancer Margaret Jeanne)* performing sketches and hosting musical acts.

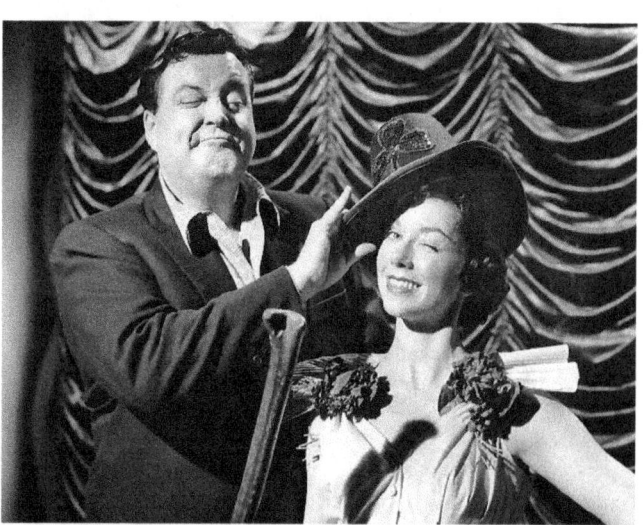

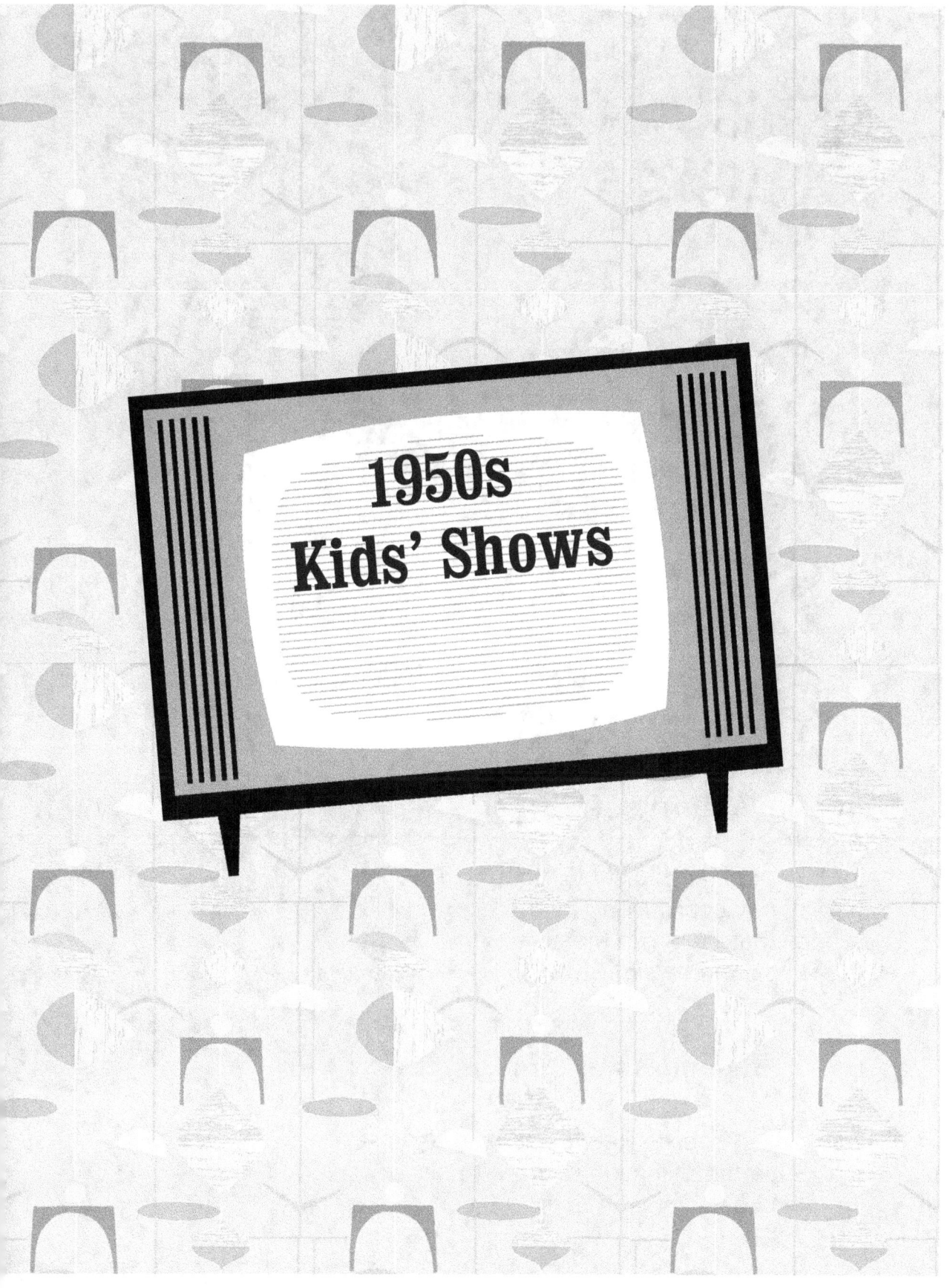

1950s
Kids' Shows

Kids' Shows

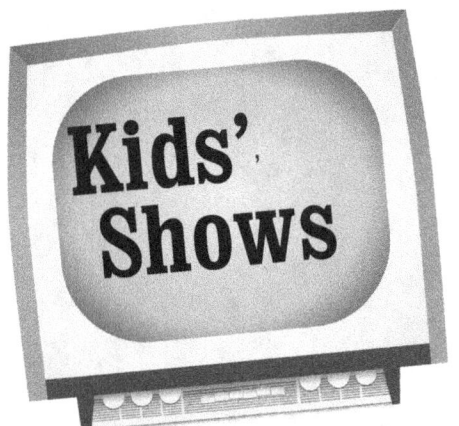

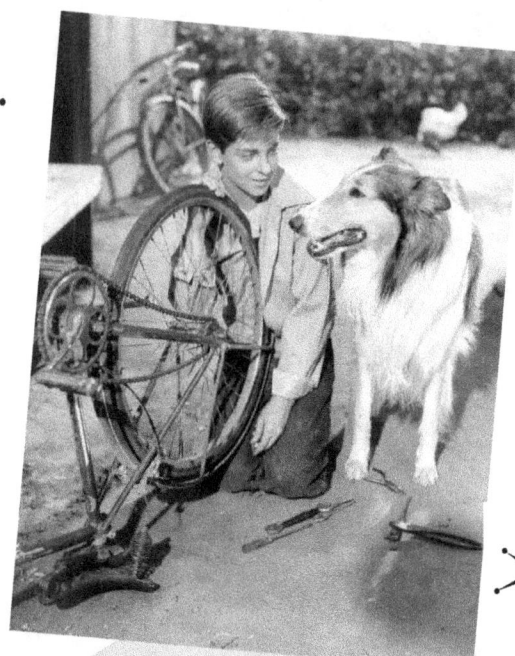

Lassie
1954-1973

This popular show was about the adventures of a collie dog, Lassie, and her young master, Jeff Miller *(above, played by Tommy Rettig).*

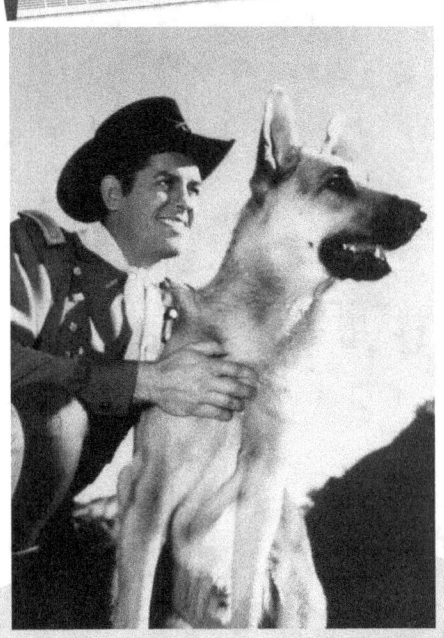

The Adventures of Rin Tin Tin
1954-1959

Another popular dog show, about US Cavalry mascot Rin Tin Tin and his owner, Lieutenant Rip Masters *(above, played by Jim Brown).*

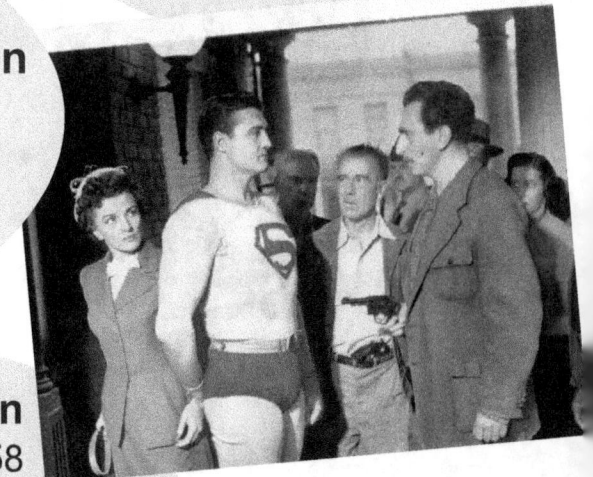

Adventures of Superman
1952-1958

George Reeves starred as Superman, fighting crime with his pals Lois Lane and Jimmy Olsen.

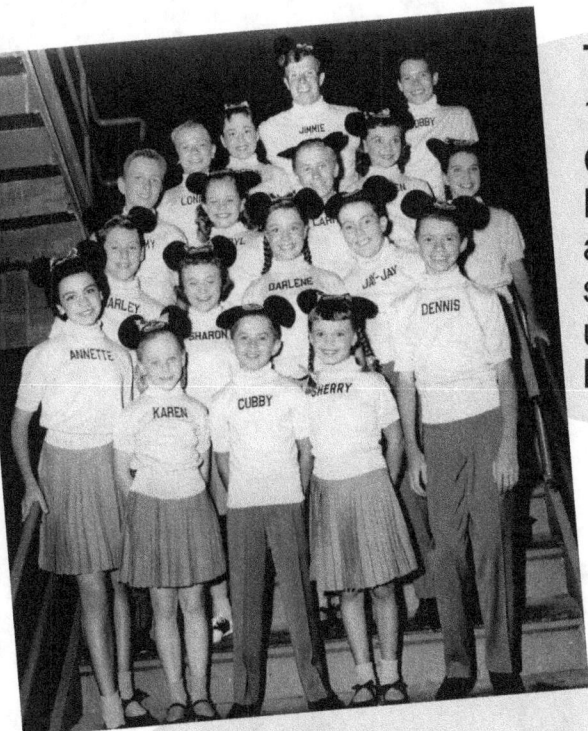

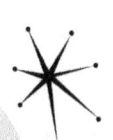

The Mickey Mouse Club
1955-1959
Club members the Mouseketeers (in Red, White and Blue teams), performed song and dance numbers under the supervision of Head Mouseketeer, Jimmie Dodd.

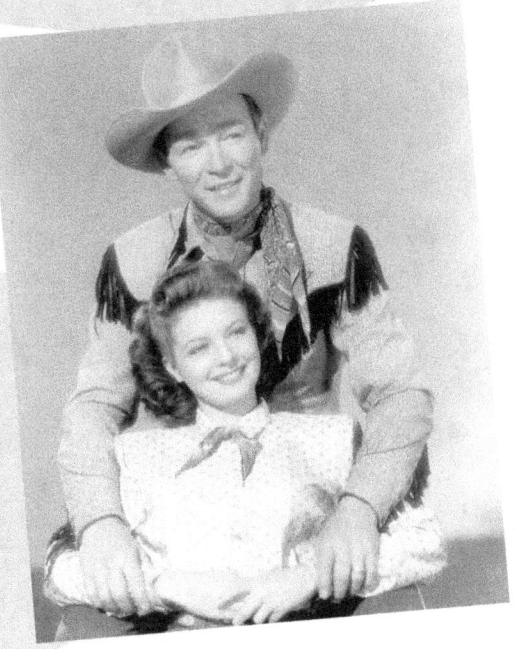

The Roy Rogers Show
1951-1957
This show was about the adventures of Roy Rogers, the singing cowboy, Trigger his golden palamino horse, and Dale Evans, Queen of the West.

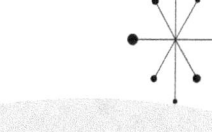

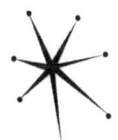

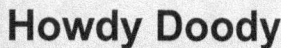

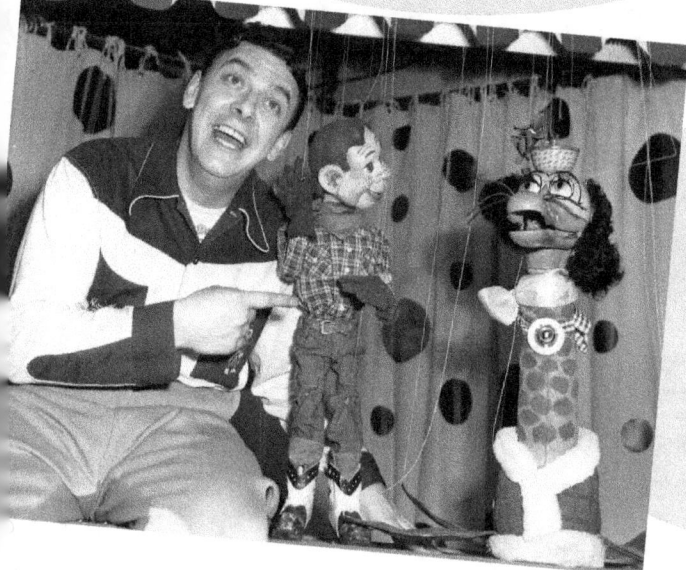

Howdy Doody
1947-1960
This show was hosted by 'Buffalo Bill' and featured cowboy puppet Howdy Doody, his sister Heidi Doody and their pet, Flub-a-Dub.

1950s Mystery and Suspense Shows

Mystery & suspense shows

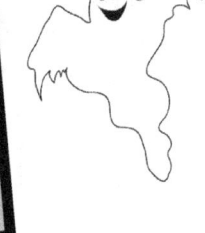

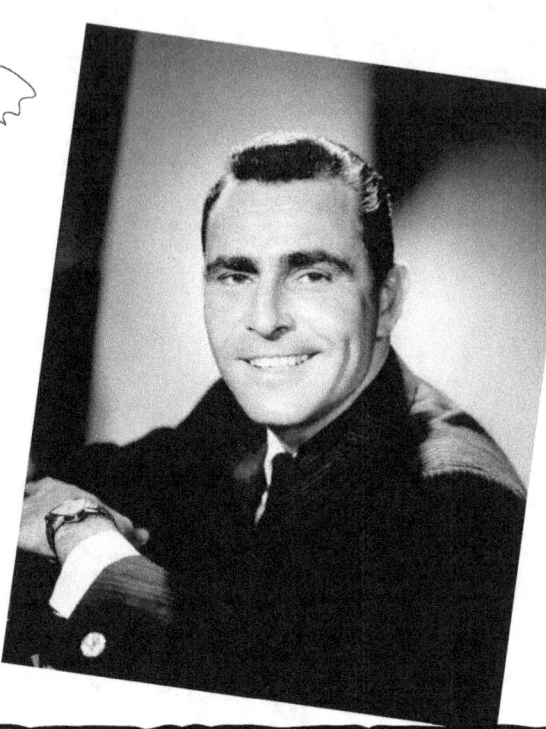

The Twilight Zone 1959-1964

Rod Serling *(right)* presented this popular show, which every week presented a tale of suspense, mystery, or science fiction, often with a supernatural twist.

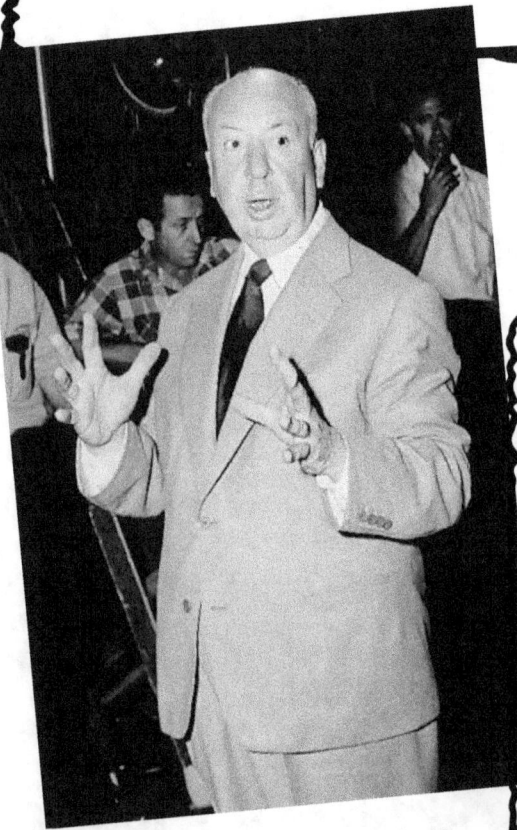

Alfred Hitchcock Presents
1955-1965

Famous movie director Alfred Hitchcock *(left)* presented this series of macabre and terrifying tales. One of the top rated shows of all time, it was shown all over the world.

One Step Beyond
1959-1961

John Newland, known as 'Your guide to the supernatural' presented this series of creepy tales on the ABC network.

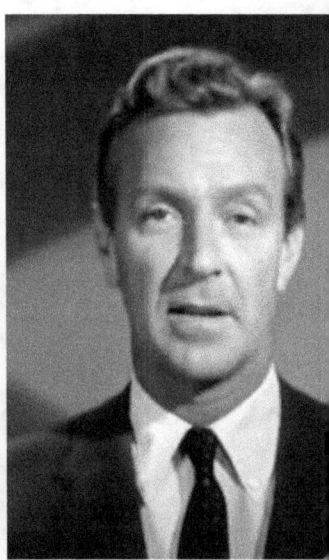

George Sanders Mystery Theater 1957

Suave British actor George Sanders *(right)* presented this series of mystery dramas which aired in the summer of 1957.

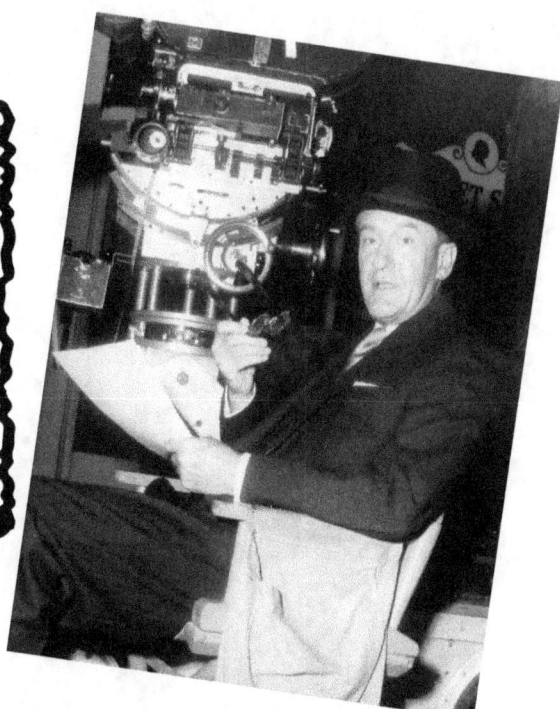

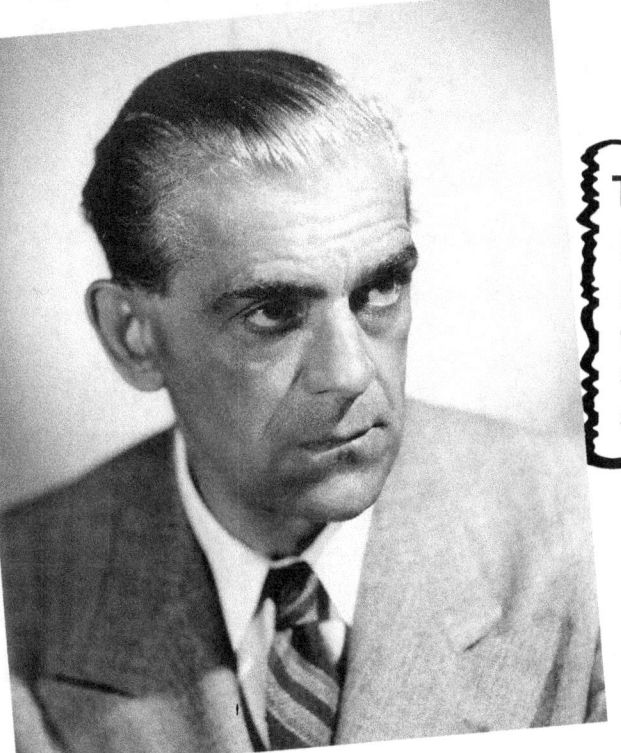

Tales of Tomorrow 1951-1953

Boris Karloff *(left)* best known for playing Frankenstein's monster, guest-starred in this series of science fiction and supernatural stories.

Lights Out 1949-1952

Vincent Price *(right)* was one of the guest stars on this series of spine-chilling dramas, based on the first US radio horror series of the same name which started in 1934.

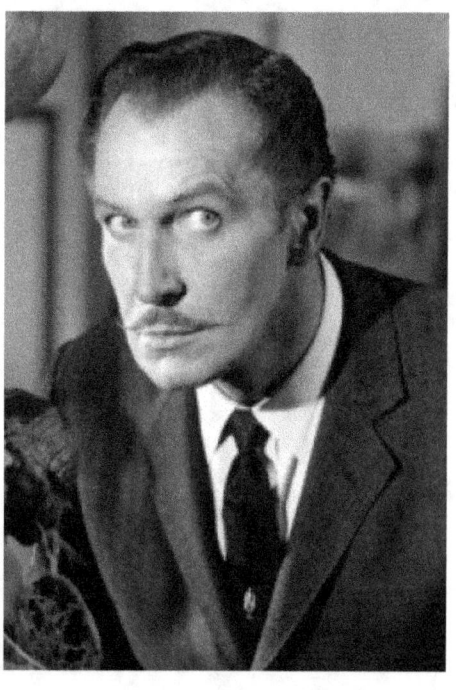

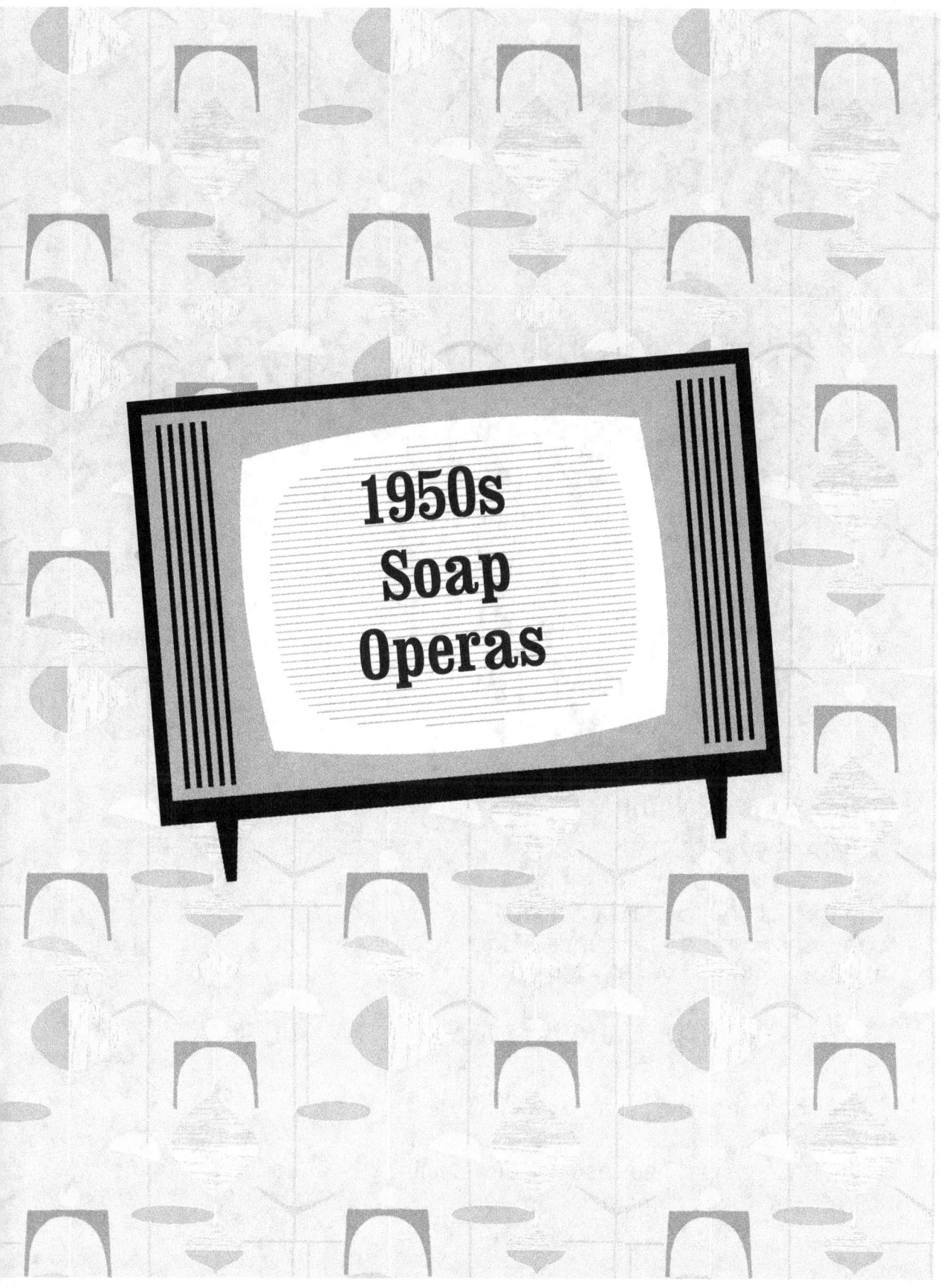

1950s
Soap
Operas

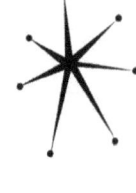

Soap operas

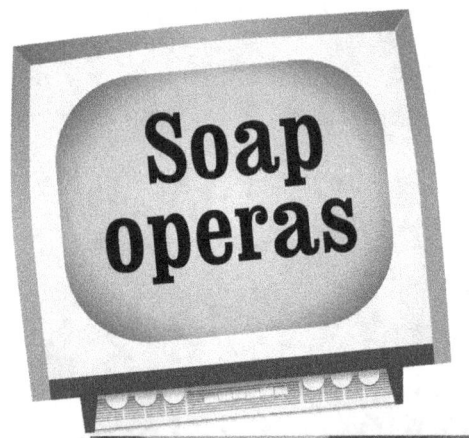

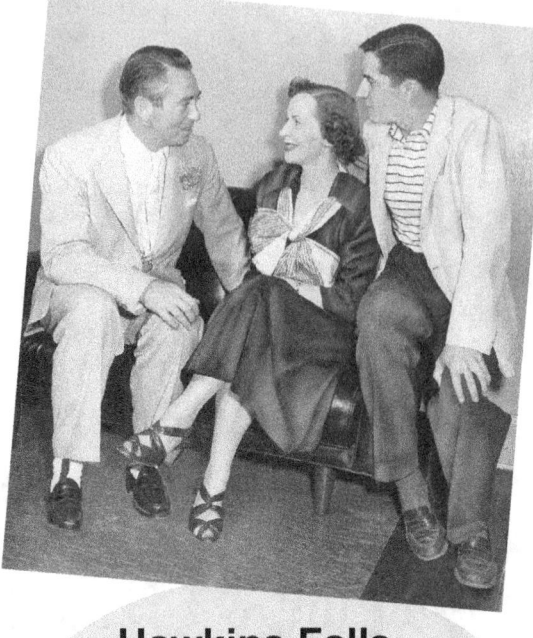

Hawkins Falls
1951-1955

This serial followed the lives of the members of the Drewer family in the small midwest town of Hawkins Falls. The show starred Bernadine Flynn *(above, with the producer and director of the show).*

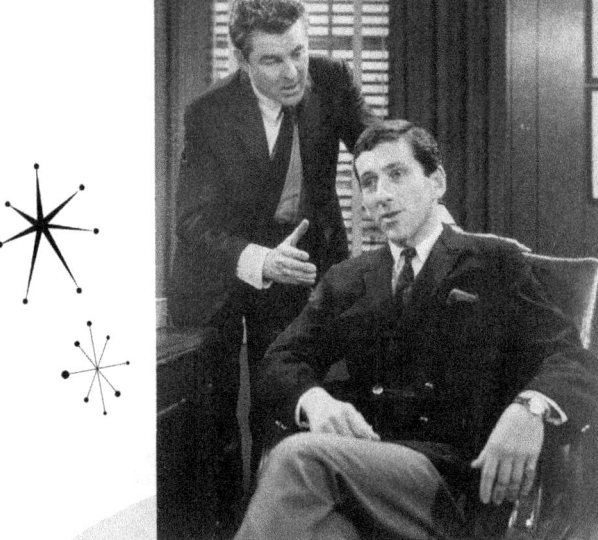

The Edge of Night
1956-1984

Set in a District Attorney's office in the fictional city of Monticello, this show starred Laurence Hugo *(above left)* as DA Mike Carr.

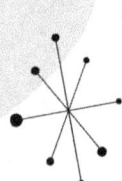

The Guiding Light
1952-2009

The longest running soap opera in TV history, this show followed the fortunes of the Bauer family. The cast included Susan Douglas Rubes *(right)* as Kathy Grant.

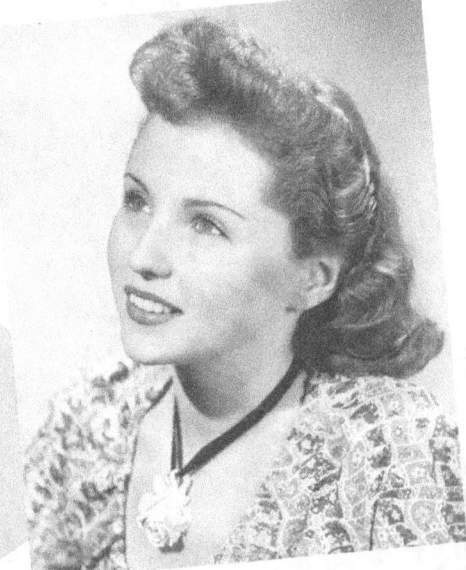

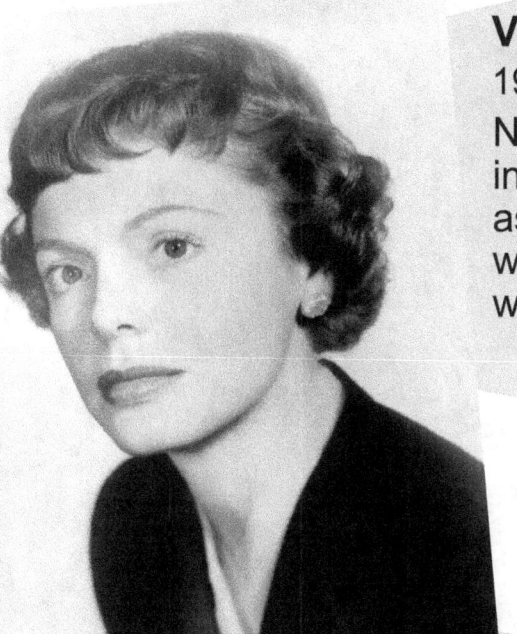

Valiant Lady
1953-1957

Nancy Coleman *(left)* starred in this CBS daily soap opera as Helen Emerson, a widow with three children, coping with the trials of life.

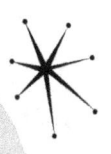

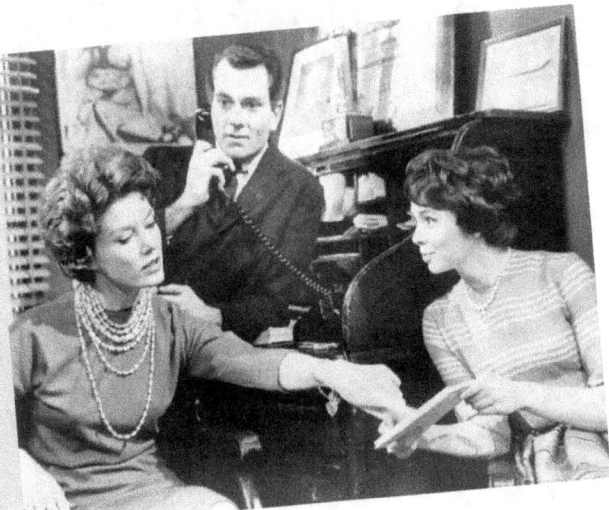

From These Roots
1958-1961

This show was about the lives and loves of the staff of a small New England family newspaper.

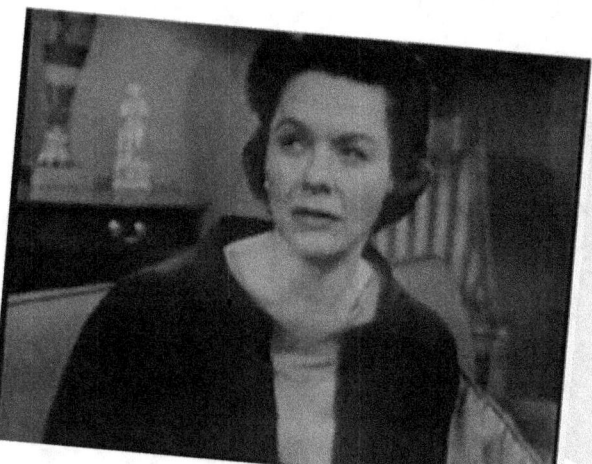

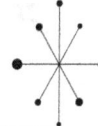

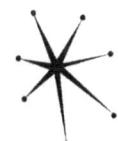

As the World Turns
1956-2010

Another long running soap opera, this show was about the personal and professional lives of a group of doctors and lawyers. It starred Helen Wagner *(left)* as Nancy Hughes McClosky.

The End

Other Memory Lane titles
Available from Amazon.com

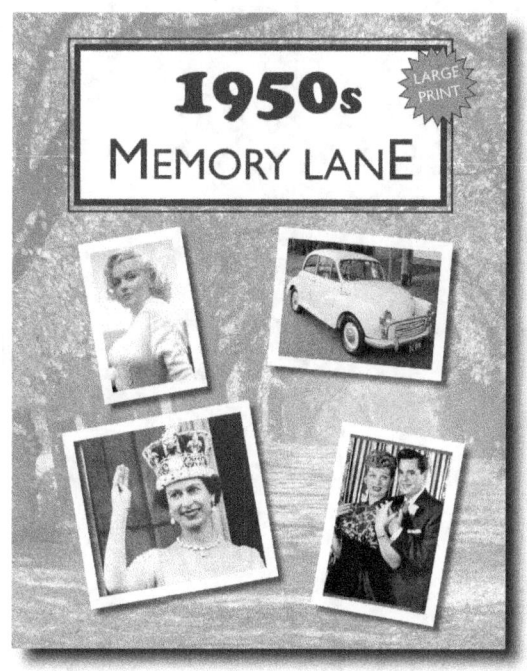

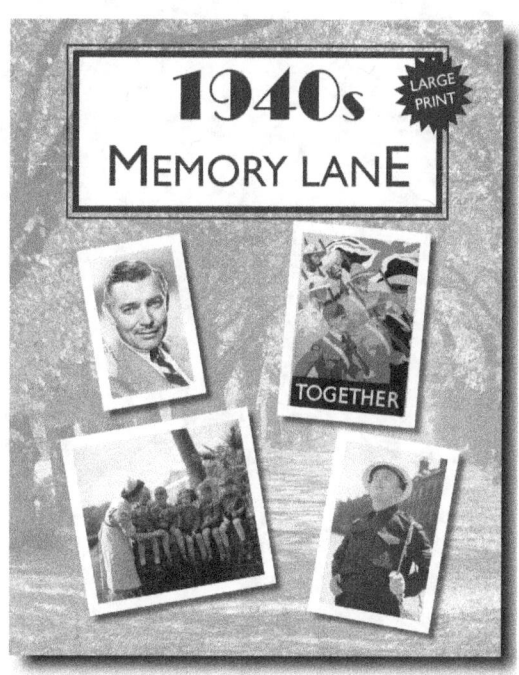

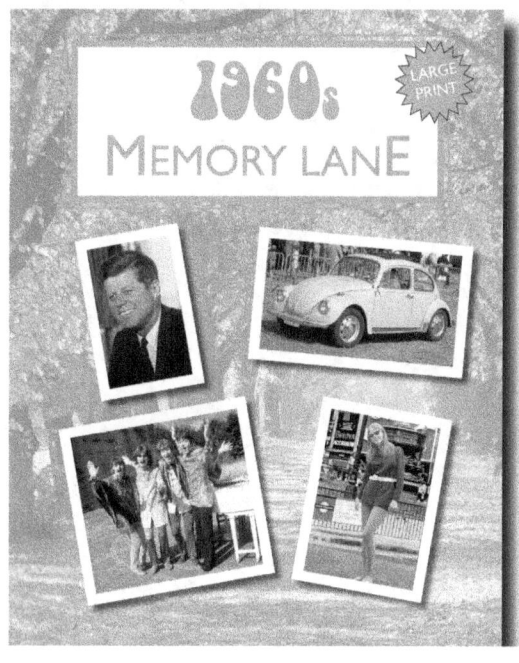

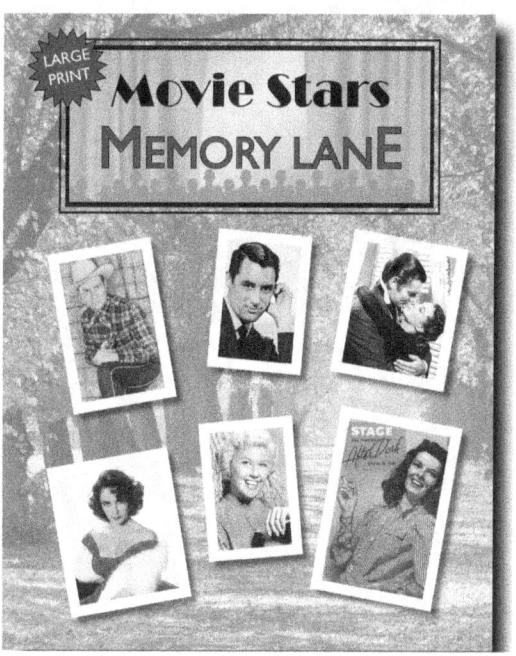